WALKING
with
GOD
through
ANXIETY AND
DEPRESSION

WALKING with GOD through ANXIETY AND DEPRESSION

A PERSONAL GUIDE

BY CHRISTIAN AUTHOR
JERALD WALL

© 2025 by Christian Author, Jerald Wall. All rights reserved.

Cover design and interior format design:
Fay Thompson, Big Moose Publishing
www.bigmoosepublishing.com

No part of this book may be reproduced or transmitted in any form without permission or consent of the author.

Disclaimer:
This book is designed to provide information and motivation to the reader. The content of this book is the sole expression and opinion of its author/publisher. You are responsible for seeking professional medical advice. The advice of the author is from his own personal experiences and should be taken as such. The author shall not be liable for any physical, psychological, emotional, financial, or commercial damages.

You are responsible for your own choices and results.

ISBN 978-0-9947995-6-2 (soft cover)
ISBN 978-0-9947995-7-9 (ebook)
Printed in Canada.

2nd edition Revised February 2025

"MY SAFE AND HAPPY PLACE IS WHEREVER I AM AT THIS VERY MOMENT."

Contents

Acknowledgments 1
Where Do You Go When the Darkness Comes? 3
Tragedies to Triumphs 5
My Testimony 7
My Story 10
What Is Anxiety? 18
What Is Depression? 23
What is Sensitization? 28
What Is Desensitization? 31
What to Remember During a Panic Attack 37
10 Steps to Your Recovery 40
Step 1: You and Your Doctor. 40
Step 2: Relaxation Techniques 46
Step 3: Positive Thinking 51
Step 4: Exposure Therapy 54
Step 5: Diet and Exercise 62
Step 6: The Power of Prayer 64
Step 7: Journaling 67
Step 8: Tear Off That Label 70
Step 9: You Have to Have Hope 73
Step 10: Your Secret Place in the Lord 76

Spiritual Warfare 79
Healing in God's Time 84
Setbacks 87
Conclusion 89
Bibliography 91
About the Author 93
Journal Pages 94

Acknowledgments

First, I want to thank God for His unending grace and love and the strength to carry on through the years.

Thank you to all the people who have helped me through the years. A special thanks to Robin Friesen, Svea Miller and Dan and Mandy Thiessen for the typing and editing.

Where Do You Go When the Darkness Comes?

Where do you go? Who do you turn to when the darkness comes? When hope fades to despair? When the world feels like it closing in around you? When you feel like you're losing your mind, losing your breath?

Your heart is racing. Your mind is racing. You feel like you're losing control. Where do you turn? Are you self-medicating yourself? Do you take drugs, alcohol, or maybe you go from bed to bed to ease the pain of how you're feeling? Perhaps you've dwelled into the occult, seeking answers, seeking hope?

You've tried everything to fix your depression, to fix your anxiety, but you're coming up short. Nothing is working and you want to give up.

While there are no easy answers in this life, may I suggest to you there is another way and His name is Jesus Christ. Where there seems to be no hope, no answers, and no way out, Jesus said, "*I am the way, the hope, and I am the life.*"

Your road to recovery starts now. It's not going to be an easy road, but no road worth traveling ever is. In this short easy to read book, I will share my steps to recovery and, looking back through many hardships, a life well lived.

May God bless you on your road to recovery.

Tragedies to Triumphs

God can take your tragedies and turn them into triumphs. That might seem hard to believe at this very moment, but it can and will happen. Your empathy for others will grow as you realize there's more to this life than the pleasures this world has to offer. Tragedies are just growing pains to the man or woman that God wants you to be. He will never let you bear more than you can handle.

In Romans 5:3-4 we read, *"Not only so, but we also glory in our sufferings, because we know that suffering produces perseverance, character and hope."*

I know from personal experience that God can turn it all around and turn your tragedies into triumphs.

My Testimony

The purpose of this book is to share my personal journey and to give hope to those who are suffering from anxiety and or depression. Though I gave my life to Jesus Christ, I rededicate my life to Him on a daily basis.

There was a time where I felt my life meant nothing. Dark clouds of depression could put me in bed for days, leaving me feeling hopeless and worthless. There was a time when anxiety and panic ravaged my mind and my body to the point where I felt I would be better dead than alive. These words sound harsh and very dramatic, but if you're reading this, you probably can relate to what I'm saying.

You might be saying to yourself right now, "Where is God when I need Him the most?…I can't find Him." "Why is this happening to me?…What did I do to deserve this?" Perhaps you are thinking of ending the suffering by leaving this world on your own… please don't! Believe it or not, God has a plan for you and for us all. Through your suffering, God will restore you and strengthen you. You will have sympathy and empathy for others that you never had before. Our God is a great God, who never breaks a promise. When He says, "I will never leave you nor forsake you," He means it!

I have realized that in my own life, I had to do my part. Don't be ashamed to reach out for help, as that is a sign of strength and not weakness. Please read the following words in this book. I pray you will find peace and encouragement.

"I know God is on my side."

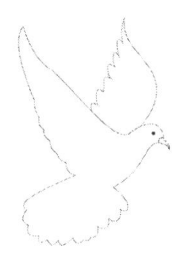

> *"I sought the LORD,
> and he answered me;
> he delivered me from
> all my fears."*
>
> *Psalm 34:4*

My Story

I was born in small town rural Saskatchewan into a wonderful Christian family of four. I'm the second youngest of the family. My siblings and I can look back on it now with laughter, but when I was a kid, things were tough for them. You see, I was labelled 'the nervous one' by my mother. My siblings couldn't touch me, because I would cause a scene by throwing a tantrum that was fear and anxiety based. I could ruin a night at the exhibition, because I could burst out into tears feeling terrified for no reason, and then we would have to pack up and go home. This was during the 1970s when there was not a lot of information on anxiety and depression. My parents did the best they could with a child that was always nervous. However, I seemed to slowly outgrow my anxieties as I got older.

In 1985, I underwent a major back surgery. Six months later, the anxiety and depression returned with a vengeance.

I still remember my first panic attack: July 2nd, 1986. I felt like I was choking, and my heart was beating out of my chest. It was absolute horror! I had no idea what was happening to me. I rushed myself to the hospital. I felt like I was having a heart attack. I was checked out by the doctor and everything was physically fine with me. They gave me something to help me relax and sent me on my way.

My life changed drastically after that. My once carefree world changed to panic attacks and depression. Every day activities became a challenge. Driving and going to work all resulted in crippling panic attacks to the point that I became housebound.

"My life has meaning."

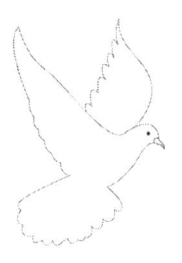

> *"Your word is a lamp for my feet, a light on my path."*
> *Psalm 119:105*

I think I felt every physical and emotional sensation a person could feel, as I will describe later on in my book. The only real place I felt safe was in the emergency room at the hospital.

Although I grew up in a Christian home, and myself had long before accepted Jesus Christ into my heart, I came to the conclusion that I had angered God or he had left me for some reason, and I was on my own to deal with this crippling affliction. When I wasn't having a panic attack, the depression would set in. A dark veil would cloud my mind for days. My world became very dark and cloudy. This would sometimes stay for days or even weeks.

After the depression lifted, the panic attacks would return. It was a vicious cycle that seemed to have no end. This went on for about two years. Then, on yet another trip to the emergency room, a doctor told me about a support group that helped people with panic and depression. This support was a Godsend. This was the beginning to my road to recovery.

"I AM NOT MENTALLY ILL."

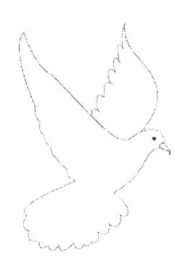

> *"So do not fear,*
> *for I am with you;*
> *do not be dismayed,*
> *for I am your God.*
> *I will strengthen you*
> *and help you;*
> *I will uphold you with*
> *my righteous right hand."*
>
> *Isaiah 41:10*

I began to understand what was happening to me and why. Through much support, information and personal prayer, my anxiety and depression began to subside and I was able to have more control over what was happening to my mind and body. My fearful dark world began to change and I started to live again without fear. The crippling panic attacks started to disappear, the depression subsided, and I started to enjoy my life again.

This was twenty five years ago, and there have been setbacks, as I will talk about later on in the book. However, through these setbacks have come renewed strength and renewed courage. Everybody's recovery will be different. Some will be longer, some will be shorter, but I assure you that you will recover.

In 2012, I lost my father. The grief was more than I could bear. The panic attacks and depression returned with a vengeance. It was as though I had forgotten everything I had learned, and my life was once more full of fear and dread. Through much prayer and coping techniques, that I will describe later in this book, I regained my life back and I became a stronger man with a greater appreciation for God and the wonderful life he has given me.

"No one has ever died from a panic attack."

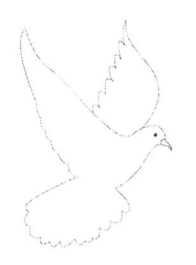

"Cast all your anxiety on Him because He cares for you."
1st Peter 5: 7

What Is Anxiety?

Anxiety is fear-based resulting in flight or fight responses. There can be many different causes of anxiety.

- **A chemical imbalance**: This is a case of when serotonin, a neurotransmitter in the brain, is below normal levels thus causing anxiety and/or depression.
- **Genetics**: Many people can trace anxiety throughout their family.
- **Substance Abuse**: Tobacco, alcohol, caffeine and others can affect serotonin levels in the brain.

- **Situational Anxiety**: One might develop anxiety during conflict in a relationship, or a work setting etc. Once the problems are resolved, the anxicty leaves as quickly as it began.
- **Social Anxiety**: A fear of interacting with others, mainly in large crowds.
- **PTSD**: Post Traumatic Stress Disorder. Mainly attributed to soldiers returning home from war, PTSD can also be applied other traumatic situations. For example: Physical or psychological abuse, motor vehicle accidents, major surgeries involving pain, suffering, and a lengthy recovery process or even an abusive relationship.
- **Agoraphobia**: When a person becomes afraid of certain situations such as open spaces, movie theatres, shopping malls etc., they start to avoid these places of perceived fear. It's easy to retreat to the safety of your home where you feel in control.

"I feel safe wherever I am."

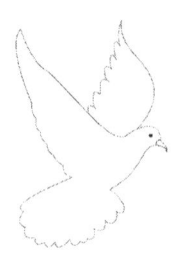

"Be strong and courageous. Do not be afraid or terrified because of them, for the LORD your God goes with you; he will never leave you nor forsake you."

Deuteronomy 31:6

There can be many different causes of anxiety. These are just a few that I have listed here. We have to be realistic; it is impossible to live in this world without some anxiety. We were born with a 'fight or flight' response mechanism. It can keep us safe. It helps us to react accordingly in dangerous situations. But if an anxiety disorder should occur, we react to dangers that aren't there. For example, you may think that an increase in your heart rate automatically means you're having a heart attack, even though your heart has been checked and is completely healthy. Another example is any strange physical sensations you may feel now means you have to run to the nearest hospital or medi-clinic.

Trust me, I know this all too well. You need to take hold and understand what is happening to you, and begin your road to recovery.

"Each day is an opportunity to learn and understand more about myself."

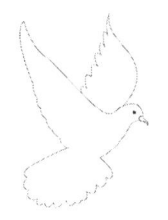

> *"Trust in the LORD with all your heart*
> *and lean not on your own understanding;*
> *in all your ways submit to Him,*
> *and He will make your paths straight."*
> *Proverbs 3: 5,6*

What Is Depression?

Depression is a state of low mood which can affect a person's well being. Feeling sad, empty, hopeless, guilty, or a sense of worthlessness are common. There can be many causes of depression. Here are some examples:

- **Biological**: Negative changes in neurotransmitter levels.
- **A Major Event**: Marriage, divorce, losing a job, losing a loved one, etc.
- **Illness**: Depression can be brought on by a medical condition.

- **Death or Loss**: Grief from a loss of a loved one is natural, but it may increase the risk of the onset of depression.
- **Conflict:** Dispute with family, friends, co-workers etc.
- **Genetics**: Some people can trace depression from their family, passed down from one generation to another.
- **Substance Abuse**: Certain drugs can cause or exacerbate depression. This can be while intoxicated or withdrawal from chronic use of drugs or alcohol.
- **SAD (Seasonal Affective Disorder)**: Reduced daylight may cause depression.
- **Situational Depression**: One might develop depression due to unmet needs, failing relationships, unsatisfying jobs or careers, etc. These issues can be resolved quickly, but some may take more time. Once the problems are resolved, the depression can subside.

"Remember, everyone experiences some form of depression on some level, from time to time."

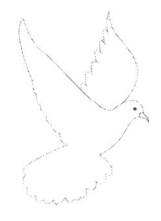

"The righteous person may have many troubles, but the LORD delivers him from them all."

Psalm 34:19

I know how devastating depression can be. It can affect every aspect of one's life. Trust me, I know from personal experience, but there's hope. Inform your doctor as there are many medications that increase the production of serotonin in the brain. Exercise can raise the endorphin levels; therefore, stimulating the neurotransmitter nor-epinephrine which is related to mood. Abstaining from drugs and alcohol will help as well, as alcohol is a depressant. Also, a sensible and healthy diet can help.

You need to get out of your bed, and you need to get out of your home and embrace life with a positive outlook. Don't give in to doubt and self pity. I've been there and it leads nowhere!

Let's not forget about prayer…God wants to help us through these trials.

"I can only live my life one day at a time."

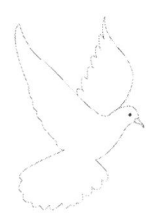

> "The LORD is a refuge for the oppressed, a stronghold in times of trouble."
> Psalm 9:9

What is Sensitization?

I had to make this as easy to understand as I could for myself and I'm going to do the same for you. Let's break this down into layman's terms. Right now, you are sensitized. You are sensitive to every thought and every feeling, and it's causing you to over-think and over-react. You're walking on eggshells. A gust of wind or the sudden blast of a horn while driving can trigger an anxiety attack. One missed heartbeat or any physical sensation can send you straight to the hospital. Perhaps you feel confused, leading you to think you're losing your mind or going crazy. I've had all these feelings tenfold. You are at the height of the fight or flight response.

Because of sensitization, you are now housebound, avoiding work, avoiding driving, avoiding crowds, or in a constant state of depression full of negative and harmful thoughts.

Now, I'm still under the assumption that you have been checked by your doctor for any underlying medical condition, so let's keep going.

As I've said before, and later in my book, the key to recovery is desensitization, and it has to start now.

"My anxiety attacks are all just waves of adrenaline. All waves subside."

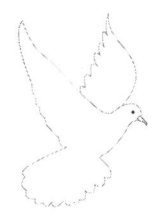

"When anxiety was great within me your consolation brought me joy."
Psalms 94:19

What Is Desensitization?

You now know that anxiety attacks almost always bring on the inevitable onset of depression, which is a state of sensitization. What now?

We desensitize ourselves!

It's not easy, but it has to be done in order for you to recover. Imagine you're afraid of heights; the very thought of climbing a ladder and walking on a rooftop may terrify you. What if one day, you climbed up the ladder, stayed a few moments and then climbed back down? The next time you climbed to the top of the ladder and stayed for a few moments and climbed back down. Now, the next time you climbed to the top, and sat on the roof with the ladder in sight, and just stayed for a few moments. Soon, you will find that each time you do this, the height becomes a little less scary. You are desensitizing yourself to the fear of heights by climbing that ladder. This is just an example of what I've done and it works.

As I will talk later in the book about exposure therapy, the key to recovery is desensitizing yourself to fearful situations. While in a panic attack, accept that nothing bad is happening to you. Don't run to the hospital because of a strange physical or emotional sensation. Of course, you have to use common sense, because there are real medical reasons for going to the hospital, but I think by now, if you're reading this book, you know what is real and what isn't... especially when you experience the same sensations every time and every time you are given a clean bill of health.

"I WILL NOT LET THIS SADNESS AND GRIEF TAKE HOLD OF ME INTO DEPRESSION."

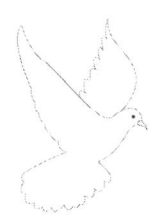

> *"When I am afraid, I put my trust in You."*
> *Psalms 56:3*

Each time you ride out your panic attack with positive thoughts and don't give in to your fears, the attacks will subside.

While in recovery, when I would have a panic attack, I would tell myself, "Okay, the doctor has given me a clean bill of health. There's nothing wrong with my heart or my lungs or anything else. I'm going to take some deep breaths and let the adrenaline flow through like a wave, and waves always subside." Sure enough, by the grace of God, each attack became less severe and held less importance.

I am at a point in my life that, when I'm faced with anxiety or some form of grief or sadness which can lead to depression, I do not let it take hold of me. I accept what is happening and realize that the wave of fear and/or the wave of sadness will subside if I let it, in order to stay desensitized.

Of course, when I talk about being desensitized, I don't mean every emotion. I simply mean fears that can seem real, but are not.

Don't be afraid to take the medications your doctor has prescribed. They have made great strides in anti-anxiety and anti-depressant medications. Use them to aid you in the desensitization process.

"I WILL CLIMB THAT LADDER OF RECOVERY ONE RUNG AT A TIME... I WILL NOT BE DISCOURAGED!"

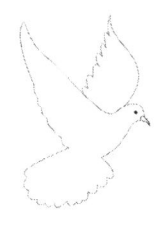

> *"He heals the broken-hearted and binds up their wounds."*
> *Psalm 147:3*

What to Remember During a Panic Attack:

- You are not going to die.
- Don't fight the attack. It's just a surge of adrenaline. It will subside in minutes if you let it.
- Don't be afraid. You are sensitized right now. The more unafraid of the attacks you become, the more desensitised you become.
- Take slow deep breaths…in through your nose and out through your mouth.

- Realize that nothing worse is going to happen to you.
- Keep reminding yourself that you have been completely checked out by your doctor. "I have a clean bill of health. These are just exaggerated feelings of stress and surges of adrenaline. I am fine."
- Remind yourself that God is in complete control.

"My anxiety attack will subside if I let it. The power is within me."

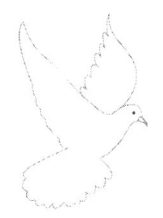

> *"The LORD will fight for you; you need only to be still."*
> *Exodus 14:14*

10 Steps to Your Recovery

Step 1: You and Your Doctor.

Anxiety can cause many emotional and physical sensations. Go to your doctor and rule out any possible health issues concerning your symptoms that you are feeling. If you have been diagnosed with anxiety and or depression, we can get started.

First, let's remember the sensations you are feeling are nothing more than your body's reaction to stress. They are neither harmful nor life threatening. No one has ever died or gone "crazy" because of an anxiety attack. These feelings can be frightening, but once you understand what is happening to you and practice the techniques I'm about to talk about, fear and hopelessness will turn to calm and confidence.

Here are some common symptoms that I and many others have experienced:

- Chest pain
- Shortness of breath
- Tingling in the hands and feet
- Feelings of unreality
- Confusion or the feeling of going "crazy"
- Racing heart
- A feeling of impending doom

These are just some of the feelings associated with anxiety. You may have other feelings or sensations, but remember they are only feelings and sensations, and nothing more. It is important to listen to your doctor. There are many different types of medication that can be very helpful. From research and my own experience, anti-depressants and other medication can be very helpful in managing anxiety and depression.

"Everyday I am getting stronger."

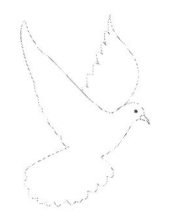

> *"But those who hope in the Lord will renew their strength. They will soar like eagles; they will run and not grow weary; they will walk and not be faint."*
>
> Isaiah 40:31

I don't want to go into great detail on the subject of taking medication, because this is between you and your doctor. Remember, if you decide to take a medication, give it time to work. I found for myself that when first taking the medication, sometimes it took a while before I felt any results.

Outside of medication, your doctor may also know of people or places that offer single or group counselling on anxiety or depression. Remember, there is no shame in taking medication for anxiety or depression any more than if you had to take medication for a headache. Don't be afraid to stay in touch with your doctor.

"I need to give my medication time to work."

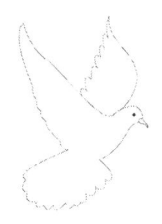

> *"Can any of you by worrying add a single hour to your life?"*
> *Matthew 6:27*

Step 2: Relaxation Techniques

There are many relaxation techniques I have used over the years. Some simple ones are a warm bath and or soothing music, but let's talk about the one I think is the most important – deep breathing.

When we are stressed, we sometimes tend to breathe too shallow or over breathe. This can lead to some unpleasant feelings such as tingling in the hands and feet, feelings of unreality, or other sensations. I want to share the breathing exercise that has worked well for me over the years. You can do this while driving or at the supermarket or wherever you are.

Take a deep breath in and counting to 4, hold for 4, breathe out for 4, and then repeat. Remember, do this nice and slow. Try to breathe through your nose and out through your mouth. If you have trouble breathing through your nose, that's okay. Breathe through your mouth nice and slow. It's very important when deep breathing to make sure you see your abdomen move up and down.

You can do this by placing one hand on your chest and one hand on your abdomen. When breathing in, you want to see your one hand on your abdomen move up and down and your hand on your chest staying as still as possible. This takes practice but you can do it.

I noticed huge improvements in my recovery doing this exercise. Your mind and your body will relax, and with enough practice, proper deep breathing will become second nature.

While you are deep breathing, meditate on the Lord. We all have a place or a word we can think of while trying to relax. Often when I'm deep breathing, on exhaling I will think the name "Jesus" as a safe word. You can use any word or thought you like. Try these techniques and see how they work for you.

"I'M GOING TO REMEMBER TO PRACTICE DEEP BREATHING WHETHER I'M ANXIOUS OR NOT!"

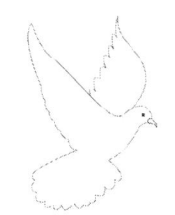

"Hear my prayer, LORD; let my cry for help come to you."
Psalm 102:1

Square Breathing Chart[1]

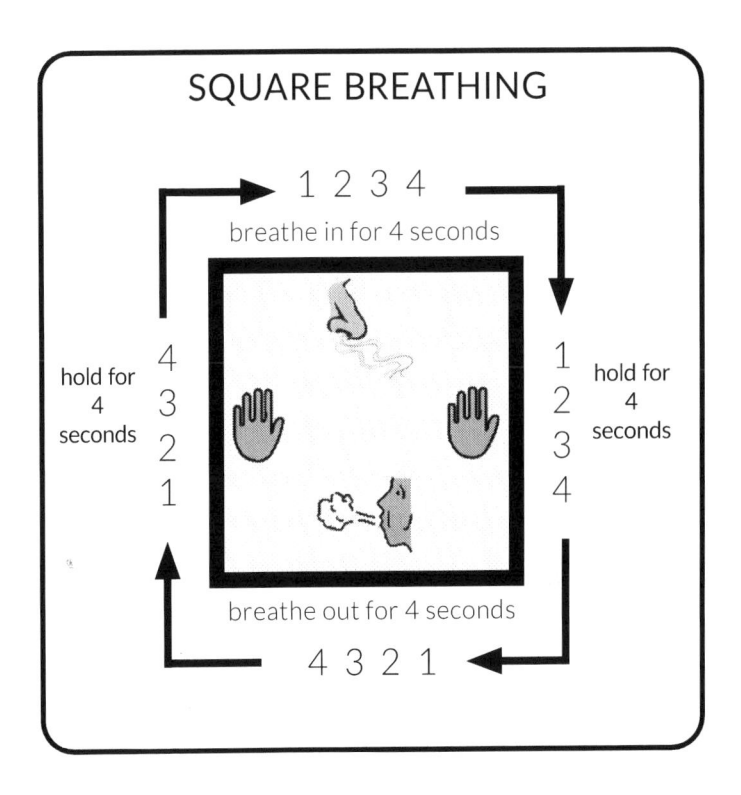

---

[1]Diagram: Elementary Counselling Blog, Wikipedia

"I'm going to practice and not test myself today."

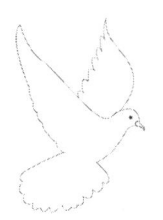

> *"Follow God's example, therefore, as dearly loved children."*
> *Ephesians 5:1*

Step 3: Positive Thinking

Positive thinking is very important. It is very easy to get caught in a vicious circle of self-defeating thinking. Such thinking as "Why can't I be normal?" or "I am mentally ill and always will be...I'll never be the person I used to be." will never lead you to peace.

Replace those thoughts with "I am not mentally ill" or "I am the same person I used to be. I'm just going through a hard time right now, but every day I'm getting better."

If you are panicking or having an anxious day, or feeling afraid, do your deep breathing and tell yourself, "I am fine. The doctor has given me a clean bill of health, and I'm just feeling sensations due to stress. These feelings will go away if I just accept them." And "I'm not going crazy. My heart is fine; my lungs are fine; it is just anxiety...plain and simple"

I can recall many times in my life when a panic attack would set me back for days or even weeks because of all the self pity and horrible things I would tell myself. I would tell myself I was worthless, and that I would never recover or be normal. I didn't realize it at the time, but every time I would talk to myself in such a way, I was sensitizing myself, putting myself in a deeper depression and delaying my recovery. It's not easy to change one's way of thinking, but it has to be done in order to recover.

Take one day at a time and trust in the Lord.

"I am not going to dwell on the negative, but instead I will focus on the positive."

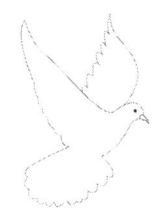

> *"Look to the LORD and His strength; seek His face always."*
> *Psalm 105:4*

Step 4: Exposure Therapy

From my own experience, this can be the most difficult step in this book. A busy line in the store, sitting in a movie theatre, driving on the highway, or maybe you're afraid to leave the safety of your own home for fear of an anxiety attack…whatever the case may be, these fearful situations CAN be overcome. It can't happen overnight, but with exposure practice, and a positive attitude, you can do it!

Let's use a few examples. If you are afraid of sitting in a crowded room or a theatre, sit near an exit, stay as long as you can. If you have to leave during the movie, don't feel defeated; remember you had the courage to go in the first place. That is a victory! You can try again. Next time you can try to sit a little longer and move a few more seats in from the aisle.

Do some deep breathing while you're sitting there. If you're having a panic attack in this situation or any other, don't be afraid to take a medication to help you to relax while you're in that panicking situation. Remember that the worst has already happened. Nothing more will happen to you. Over time you will be able to sit through an entire movie. This can apply to standing in line in the store or other fearful situations.

I used to have horrible panic attacks at the movie theatre. I spent most of my time in the bathroom or lobby instead of watching the movie. The fight or flight response at that time was at its peak. Although the movie theatre was a place of fear for me, I kept going back and tried to sit a little longer each time, instead of running to the bathroom or lobby. I didn't realize it at the time, but I was desensitizing myself by returning and sitting as long as I could.

"There are wonderful things in store for me."

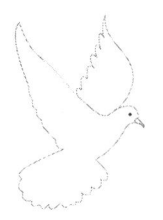

> *"Call to me and I will answer you and show you great and mighty things which you do not know."*
> *Jeremiah 33:3*

I can recall driving one block and would have to pull over because my heart was racing. I had a feeling of shortness of breath, and I would drive home or straight to the hospital.

After a clean bill of health, the next day I pressed on and kept driving. The symptoms would return, but I didn't rush home or to the hospital. I would pull over, take some deep breaths, accept what was happening to me, tell myself that I had just had a clean bill of health from the doctor and sure enough, the symptoms would start to subside. I was not going to be defeated by irrational fears.

If you have a fear of driving on the highway, go for short trips. Have it in mind that if you need to turn around, you won't be discouraged. Remember it is a victory just to get into the car and try. Remember each mile, each block, each step is a victory. When you start to desensitize yourself, you gain strength in mind and body. Situations you once found fearful start to become less so, and things become easier to do.

I want to share some words from Dr. Claire Weekes, a wonderful general practitioner and health writer. Her four steps to overcoming anxiety are:

1. **Face** - Face what makes you afraid. Don't fight it because this will trigger more adrenaline and worsen your condition.

2. **Accept** - Accept what is happening to you without fear, thus reducing the triggering of adrenaline.

3. **Float** - Float through the fear with calm.

4. **Let time pass** - Allow yourself time to fully recover; time will heal.

I have relied on these steps many times in my life and found them essential in recovery.

"I will not compare my progress with someone else's...I am recovering and that's all that matters."

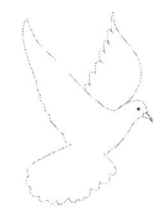

> "Is anyone among you in trouble? Let them pray. Is anyone happy? Let them sing songs of praise."
>
> James 5:13

As in every fearful situation, you keep trying. Each time you get in the car and drive a little farther, you desensitize yourself. The same can be applied for example, if you find it hard to leave the safety of your home.

Start with walks around the block. Watch the people around you; remember you are not mentally ill. You are just sensitized and you will overcome your difficulties. If you have to turn around and go home, that's okay. Don't be discouraged, you will try again tomorrow.

Don't compare your progress to someone else's as each person desensitizes themselves in their own time. Don't put pressure on yourself, and don't test yourself…just practice! Remember there was a time when I couldn't leave the safety of my own home, except to go to a hospital. With small steps, I practiced these techniques and now make trips to the mountains, sit through movies, and stand in busy shopping lines. I promise you; it can be done!

"If I am having a bad day in my recovery, I'm still always moving forward…never backward."

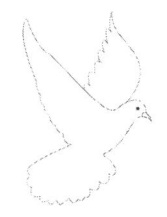

"Therefore confess your sins to each other and pray for each other so that you may be healed. The prayer of a righteous person is powerful and effective."
James 5:16

Step 5: Diet and Exercise

Exercising is very important. Studies show that regular exercise release endorphins that can improve and stimulate the production of serotonin in the brain. In my opinion, this is essential in the maintaining of mood levels thus reducing anxiety and depression. Exercise can strengthen your immune system, keeping your body and mind healthy, and keep at bay, many physical ailments such as heart disease, diabetes, arthritis etc.

Have you heard the phrase "you are what you eat"? This is certainly true in my case. I was a sugar addict, and my body and my mind know how destructive this was for me and how much it fed my depression and panic disorder. It was only after I limited my sugar intake and realized the harmful effects of alcohol, tobacco, and caffeine that I saw a huge reduction in my panic attacks and depression. Alcohol is a depressant that only worsened my mood. Caffeine is a stimulant that triggered my panic attacks. You know your body. Talk to your doctor in regards to exercise and your own personal diet.

"I'm going to trust in God, and lay my troubles at his feet."

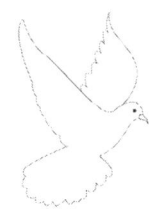

> *"In peace I will lie down and sleep, for you alone, LORD, make me dwell in safety."*
> *Psalm 4:8*

Step 6: The Power of Prayer

Do not underestimate the power of prayer. It is a direct line to God himself. Day or night, He is there for you. He does not get tired of you. It doesn't cost you a thing. The Lord says in James 5:16, *"Confess your faults one to another, and pray one for another, that ye may be healed. The effectual fervent prayer of a righteous man availeth much."*

Never give up, your prayers are always heard. God answers in His time. Pray with all your heart, always giving Him praise and thanks for what He has done for you, and what He will do for you. Remember others as well. There is always somebody in a worse situation than you or I are in.

God loves you and always wants to be in contact with you. Please make time for Him. Remember in Philippians 4:6,7 these words:

"Do not be anxious about anything, but in every situation, by prayer and petition, with thanksgiving, present your requests to God."

"And the peace of God, which transcends all understanding, will guard your hearts and your minds in Christ Jesus."

Also, in 1st John 5:14 *"This is the confidence we have in approaching God: that if we ask anything according to his will, he hears us."*

"I am not losing control or going crazy."

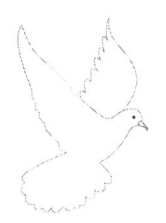

> *"Heal me, LORD, and I will be healed; save me and I will be saved, for you are the one I praise."*
>
> Jeremiah 17:14

Step 7: Journaling

I found that writing down my thoughts while having a panic attack or while I was in a state of depression, I could see how irrational my thoughts really were. Write down what you're feeling at that very moment, and then write down something positive that you know to be true. Be sure to date it to keep track of your progress.

Example One:

December 5th, 2015

Fear: I'm feeling short of breath and my heart is racing.

I am terrified!

Response: I have been checked out by the doctor and my heart and lungs are fine. This is just a surge of adrenaline, there's nothing wrong with me.

Example Two:

December 10th, 2015

Fear: I feel so sad; I don't want to get out of bed today.

Response: I'm going to get out of bed and do something productive, because my life has meaning.

Writing down your fears, and then a positive affirmation seemed to really benefit me. I could see on paper just how irrational my thoughts really were. At the end of this book, I'm leaving empty pages for you to try on your own. I think you'll really benefit from it. Good luck.

"I will not give in to irrational fears."

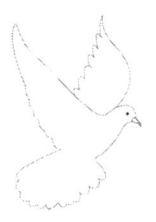

> *"My help comes from the LORD, the Maker of heaven and earth."*
> *Psalm 121:2*

Step 8: Tear Off That Label

At some point in our lives, we are usually labelled by ourselves or others. We can be labelled as kind or unkind, a hard worker or someone who slacks on the job. The label that has defined your life and how you live it is the one that has to be removed.

I was labelled as a nervous person at a young age, and for many years I lived that way even when I wasn't nervous or depressed at all. Since I had that attached to me, that's how I lived. Though anxiety and depression may fall under that mental illness umbrella, I found it essential to remove that "nervous person" label.

Carrying a label around with you can keep you in a constant state of anxiety and depression just on its own. It can become a self-fulfilling prophecy that will keep you down as long as you let it. I changed my label from a "nervous person" to "I'm as normal as anyone else, and harsh words will not define my life." God defines my life and nothing else. I encourage you to replace your label with a positive one, and start your road to recovery.

As I said at the beginning of the book in 'My Story', I came from a wonderful Christian home and my parents did their very best with a child with a nervous condition.

I wouldn't trade my childhood or how I was raised for anything. Labels can be attached very innocently as was in my case.

"MY OLD LABEL IS GONE. I HAVE REPLACED IT WITH A POSITIVE ONE."

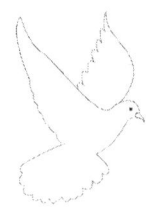

"He who began a good work in you will carry it on to completion until the day of Christ Jesus."

Philippians 1:6

Step 9: You Have to Have Hope

What is hope? Billy Graham, the great evangelist stated in his book, "The reason for my hope, God has made the plan of redemption plain. Finding Jesus Christ and having the assurance of His salvation is essential to securing eternal life with Him in Heaven."

You see, when we come to the realization that this life is all about Him, and it's all for Him, and our salvation is secured, then and only then will we find hope and strength in our lives. Your afflictions, though difficult, will strengthen you not only to recover, but to become someone more that you thought you could ever be. I became a prayer warrior, empathising with others in their struggles, and an evangelist who yearns to share the gospel of Jesus Christ to anyone who will listen. I have hope and strength, through the trials I have been through, not of myself, but of my Lord Jesus Christ.

How can we have hope in our lives, if we have no hope in our salvation? I know that my life would have no meaning without Jesus first. We have to deal with and secure our faith in Christ and then everything else will fall in to place.

"Every morning I pray for hope."

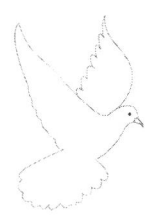

> *"The righteous will inherit the land and dwell in it forever."*
> *Psalm 37:29*

Step 10: Your Secret Place in the Lord

Psalm 91[1]

[1] Whoever dwells in the shelter of the Most High will rest in the shadow of the Almighty.

[2] I will say of the LORD, "He is my refuge and my fortress, my God, in whom I trust."

[3] Surely He will save you from the fowler's snare and from the deadly pestilence.

[4] He will cover you with his feathers, and under his wings you will find refuge; his faithfulness will be your shield and rampart.

[5] You will not fear the terror of night, nor the arrow that flies by day,

[6] nor the pestilence that stalks in the darkness, nor the plague that destroys at midday.

[7] A thousand may fall at your side, ten thousand at your right hand, but it will not come near you.

---

[1] https://www.biblegateway.com/passage/?search=Psalm+91&version=NIV#fen-NIV-15397a

⁸ You will only observe with your eyes and see the punishment of the wicked.

⁹ If you say, "The LORD is my refuge," and you make the Most High your dwelling,

¹⁰ no harm will overtake you, no disaster will come near your tent.

¹¹ For He will command His angels concerning you to guard you in all your ways;

¹² they will lift you up in their hands, so that you will not strike your foot against a stone.

¹³ You will tread on the lion and the cobra; you will trample the great lion and the serpent.

¹⁴ "Because he loves me," says the LORD, "I will rescue him; I will protect him, for he acknowledges my name.

¹⁵ He will call on me, and I will answer him; I will be with him in trouble, I will deliver him and honor him.

¹⁶ With long life I will satisfy him and show him my salvation."

"I put my complete faith in God and in Him alone."

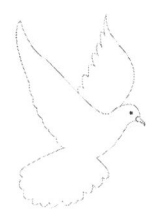

"Then the eyes of the blind shall be opened, and the ears of the deaf shall be unstopped."

Isaiah 35:5

Spiritual Warfare

As I've talked about earlier, we all get sad, depressed or anxious from time to time; we're human, it's natural. However, when anxiety and depression last so long, with panic raging on a daily basis, and the kind of depression that keeps a person in bed for days, weeks, even months, you become another person. At least, that's how it was for me. It was as though I wasn't in charge of myself anymore, or perhaps something else was. After I figured out what was happening to me, I knew I had an emotional problem, not a spiritual one.

I have counselled people who have let things into their lives that they shouldn't have. You see, there is a constant battle waging for your soul. As a Christian, I don't believe you can become possessed; however, I do believe you can become oppressed. You see, some people will seek alternative solutions not realizing that when dealing with the spirit realm, you are dealing with either God or Satan, no in between! Satan does not want to help you; it's quite the opposite. He hates you and wants to destroy your life. Perhaps there might be a short term of relief playing with Satan, but it will come at a cost. Ultimately your situation will worsen, and you will have to deal with that open demonic door.

"I will trust in God only."

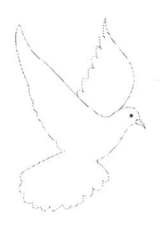

> *"Whom resists steadfast in the faith, knowing that the same afflictions are accomplished in your brethren that are in the world."*
>
> *1st Peter 5:9*

The Bible is very clear about what God thinks about consulting spirits through ouija boards, tarot cards, psychics etc. In Leviticus, Chapter 19:31 God says, "*Regard not them that have familiar spirits neither seek after wizards or to be defiled by them: I am the Lord your God.*" Also in 1st Peter 5:8 "*Be sober, be vigilant; because your adversary, as a roaring lion, walketh about, seeking whom he may devour.*"

Once that door is opened, you give the enemy power that is greater than your own. Was this me? No! By the grace of God I never went down that path. Is it you? I am certainly not saying that your anxiety or depression are a result of this; however, if you have opened the door to that demonic spirit realm, you need to close it. Only God can do that by asking Him through prayer. In James 2:19, "*Thou believest that there is one God; thou doest well: the devils also believe and tremble. I am the LORD your God.*"

"With God's help I can discern what is right and what is wrong."

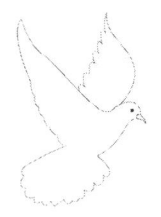

> "May my prayer come before you; turn your ear to my cry."
> Psalm 88:2

Healing in God's Time

I know when we are suffering, we want healing right now. Unfortunately it doesn't always work that way. When we have faith in the Lord, healing can come right away or it can be a process. In my case it was a process. A healing process of much prayer, time, patience and help from health care professionals. In Psalm 27:14, God says, "*Wait on the Lord: be of good courage. He shall strengthen thine heart: wait, I say, on the Lord.*" I want to share the words to a hymn written many years ago by John H. Sammis in 1887 called 'Trust and Obey'.

Not a shadow can rise,
not a cloud in the skies
But His smile quickly drives it away;

Not a doubt or a fear,
not a sigh or a tear,
Can abide while we trust and obey.

Don't these words say it all? We must trust and obey in our Lord.

"I'm going to work in God's timetable and not my own."

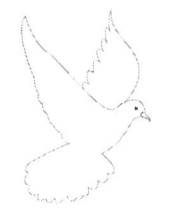

> *"When the time is right, I the Lord will make it happen."*
> *Isaiah 60:22*

Setbacks

I've had many setbacks through the years, but with each setback came new strength and new courage. I look at it as an opportunity to practice techniques that I've used in the past that have worked for me, and I hope they will work for you. Setbacks can give you a renewed sense of the blessings that you have in your life, and that we should never forget.

Each setback, for me, became shorter and shorter because of the knowledge I had gained through the experience and process of these steps that I have shared with you in this booklet.

"My doctor has given me a clean bill of health. There is nothing physically or mentally wrong with me."

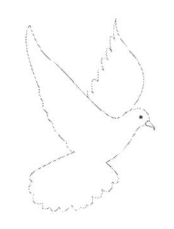

"Praise the LORD, my soul, and forget not all His benefits who forgives all your sins and heals all your diseases."

Psalm 103: 2, 3

Conclusion

I know what you're going through. A panic attack is a terrifying experience. Depression sets in like a sad and dark veil that refuses to lift. I'm here to tell you that the anxiety will subside and that dark veil will lift. God is not angry with you. He has not left you or forsaken you. You are not going crazy; you're not mentally ill; and, you're going to recover.

Remember:

- Go to your doctor.
- If instructed, take medication and give it time to work.

- Seek out counselling.
- Expose yourself to the things that frighten you. Through exposure you will desensitize yourself.
- Ride out panic attacks like a wave... waves always subside.
- Don't hide in depression. Embrace life with a positive attitude.
- Eat healthy and live a clean lifestyle.
- Stay away from the occult. Nothing but grief and sorrow will come from that.
- Trust in God; He loves you!

I think sometimes we have to endure troubles to appreciate the blessings God has given to us. Through this experience I have realized the greatness of our Lord. You do not have to go through this alone. Stay the course, and if you haven't already, I encourage you to accept Jesus into your life.

I hope that this book will encourage you and help keep you on track...and keep fighting the good fight and never give up! God Bless!

Bibliography

New International Version Bible (NIV), Zondervan Publishing, 2019.

Holy Bible, New King James Version, Thomas Nelson; Lea edition, 2018.

KJV Holy Bible, Thomas Nelson; Gift edition, 2017.

Dr. Claire Weekes, Hope and Help for Your Nerves, Berkley Books, 1990.

Billy Graham, The Reason for My Hope, W Publishing Group, Nashville, Tennessee, 2013.

John H. Sammis, Trust and Obey, https://library.timelesstruths.org/music/Trust_and_Obey/, 1887.

About the Author

Through the grace of God, Jerald wall was able to recover from severe anxiety and depression, and now lives a life full of gratitude, helping others to do the same.

Jerald holds a diploma in Psychology and Social Work from Stratford Career Institute (2023), a certificate from the Billy Graham School of Evangelism (2019), and a certificate in General Counselling and Guidance from Granton Institute of Technology (2005).

To learn more about Jerald and his work, visit:

facebook.com/jeraldwallministries
instagram.com/welcomejerald1968
youtube.com/@jeraldwallministries2637
tiktok @jeraldwallministries
rumble.com/user/jeraldwallministries

Journal Pages

Journal Pages

Journal Pages

Journal Pages

Journal Pages

Journal Pages

Journal Pages

Journal Pages

Journal Pages

Manufactured by Amazon.ca
Bolton, ON